THE PREVENTION IMPERATIVE

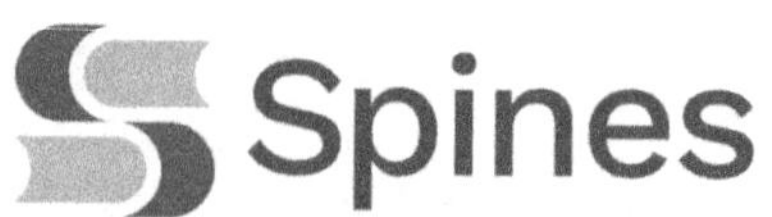

THE PREVENTION IMPERATIVE

THE SIMPCO SOLUTION: BETTER HEALTHCARE OUTCOMES FOR AMERICA

JEFFREY STERLING, MD, MPH

IN COLLABORATION WITH
CAROL ADAMS, PHD

AND

NIVA LUBIN-JOHNSON, MD

CONTENTS

INTRODUCTION

I recall having an "I'm still alive and avoided becoming a statistic" birthday party when I turned twenty-five years old. In many ways, that was much more of a statement of reality than a reflection of sentimentality. There are conditions across America that subject citizens of various demographic and geographic considerations to increased risk and incidence of worse healthcare outcomes than the general population. Consider the following examples.

- An analysis of the top 10 zip codes in Chicago suffering deaths during the COVID-19 pandemic showed residents of predominantly Black and Latinx populations suffered almost three times the number of mortalities as did those in the top ten suffering White communities.[1]
- According to the National Institutes of Health (NIH), male coal miners in southern West Virginia are at increased risk of cancer, heart failure, ischemic heart disease, and mental health disorders.[2]

- The NIH also notes that rural Americans are more likely to die prematurely from leading causes of death, including heart disease, cancer, lung disease, and stroke. They suffer from higher rates of obesity and diabetes and are at greater risk of fatal motor vehicle crashes, suicides, and drug overdoses.[3]
- Across twenty-four measures, Mississippi ranked near the bottom or last among states when measuring health outcomes, healthcare access, and healthcare quality. These outcomes included the lowest life expectancy, the highest infant death rate, and one of the highest maternal death rates in the country.[4]

Now, consider the effect of the above on the quality of your life if you just happen to be a part of any of those demographics. Although geographically specific, these statistics -examples of healthcare disparities- aren't isolated findings as much as representations of unique, situational expressions of fault lines, representing challenges within the US healthcare system. When these challenges are simply the result of where and how you live, they are described as social determinants of health.

An irony of the US healthcare system is there are tremendous financial resources expended on health and medical care, yet these challenges and disparities exist and persist in a variety of ways for a variety of communities across America. However, there are opportunities to be found. Best practices do exist that, if implemented, would improve overall performance within the system, and they would address, at least in part, the above examples and many more like them.

CHAPTER ONE

HEALTHCARE DISPARITIES AND SOCIAL DETERMINANTS OF HEALTH

Social influencers and determinants of health (SDOH) have a major impact on people's health, well-being, and quality of life. SDOHs focus on causes. These differences exist because of a broad variety of characteristics, including the following:[5]

- Age
- Disability status
- Economic status
- Environment
- Ethnicity
- Gender
- Geographic location
- Race
- Sexual Orientation

Health disparities refer to higher burdens of illnesses, injuries, or mortality experienced by a group relative to others. Healthcare disparities refer to differences in health coverage, access to care, and quality of care between groups. When describing these disparities, the focus is on outcomes. They signify lesser health for those affected. They reflect a diminished ability to function and a reduced quality of life. They indicate increased risks for disease and death.

Health disparities are linked to social determinants of health. Their persistence reflects flaws within the design and implementation of healthcare systems, and they represent challenges toward having a level of quality of life for those affected. Eradicating healthcare disparities is a major consideration in the Healthy People 2030 goals.[5]

Consider the following 2021 life expectancy data from the National Center for Health Statistics, covering the general population and selected racial and ethnic groups.[6]

- Asian Total: 83.5 years
- All Females: 79.3 years
- Hispanic Total: 77.8 years
- White Total: 76.7 years
- General Population Total: 76.4 years
- All Males: 73.5 years
- Black Total: 71.2 years
- American Indian and Alaska Native (AIAN) Total: 65.6 years

The above data shows Asians, females, and White Americans have higher life expectancies than the general population, and males, Black Americans and AIAN citizens have lower life expectancies. A resulting ongoing policy discussion and set of decisions involve whether incremental public health efforts are better spent increasing the life expectancy for the entire population or by focusing on uplifting those populations that suffer years below the norm (i.e., have health disparities). As another example, using the same data, Black females have a life expectancy at birth of 75.0 years, whereas Black males have a life expectancy of 67.6. It's reasonable to conclude in this example, and others like it, targeted health initiatives would be in order. Of course, with the amount of money being spent on healthcare in the US, the choices aren't mutually exclusive, but the data provide important facts on failures, needs, and opportunities for improvement within the system and for its population.

Of course, increasing life expectancies involves both looking at the causes of death and the conditions increasing the risks of death. Reasonable efforts to address the causes of death would prioritize looking at the most common causes of death, along with identifying the most preventable causes of death.

Here are the top five causes of death in the US for 2021.[7]

1. COVID-19
2. Heart Disease
3. Malignant neoplasms (cancers)
4. Accidents (intentional injuries)
5. Cerebrovascular disease

Now, here are the top causes of death for different ethnicities for 2021.[7]

- American Indians and Alaska Natives: COVID-19
- Asians: Malignant neoplasms
- Blacks: Heart disease
- Hispanics: COVID-19
- Whites: Diseases of the heart

According to the Centers for Disease Control and Prevention (CDC), the five leading causes of preventable early deaths are heart disease, cancer, unintentional injury, chronic lower respiratory disease, and stroke. Another example of healthcare disparities is found here. These early deaths are more common among people living in rural communities compared to Americans who live in urban areas.[8]

As a policy imperative, the CDC addresses ways healthcare practitioners can help prevent premature deaths. They include the following.

- Screen patients for high blood pressure.
- Increase cancer prevention and early detection.
- Encourage physical activity and healthy eating.
- Treat opioid use disorder.
- Help patients quit smoking.

Unfortunately, simply identifying and targeting the management of preventable premature deaths isn't sufficient to address all that's involved in preventable mortality. Each entity causing death has distinct risk factors and requires nuanced prevention and medical strategies.

However, across most efforts to prevent and manage disease and promote health, several challenges seem to be consistent, and they present as healthcare disparities. These factors are often cited as emblematic of the challenges facing the American healthcare system.

They include the following:

- Access to care.
- Cost of care.
- Presence of social factors contributing to disease.
- Varying incidences and impacts of various diseases between communities.
- Differing adverse health outcomes between communities.

It bears reemphasizing that each of these considerations is a social determinant of health. More formally, social determinants of health (SDOH) are the conditions in the environments where people are born, live, learn, work, play, worship, and age that affect a wide range of health, functioning, and quality-of-life outcomes and risks.[5] To fully address preventable mortality, identifying and addressing the social determinants of health is an ongoing requirement. Here are a few examples of SDOH.

Safe housing, transportation, and neighborhoods:

- Homes across America are subject to mold, cat and other animal dander that cause allergies. Insect bites cause infections and other disease. Exposed electrical wires cause burns and other trauma. Your home could literally be making you sick.

- Imagine if you live in a community with inadequate public and private transportation. How exactly do you get to work and provide for your family? How promptly can you get to a hospital in the midst of a stroke or heart attack when seconds matter? This reality for many Americans is as important of a contributor to health as being screened, diagnosed, and treated for an illness.

- What if your neighborhood is afflicted with high crime and violence rates or is in the midst of toxic chemicals? What if you live in regions afflicted by hurricanes or tornados in an ongoing manner? The increased health risks and causes of death are foreseeable.

Racism, discrimination, and violence:

- The ways racism and discrimination impact health are numerous. Institutional racism results in poorer access to care, higher costs of care, and lesser quality of care. An often-cited example of discrimination in medical treatment is the systemwide administration of smaller doses of pain medication for the same clinical situations in Black patients than for others in the general population.[9]

- There are also well-known examples of healthcare outcomes that display systemic discrimination in clinical practice. For example, non-Hispanic Blacks/African Americans have a 2.4 times higher infant mortality rate than non-Hispanic whites. Maternal mortality rates for non-Hispanic Blacks are 2.6 times the rate for non-Hispanic White women.[10,11] In fact, Black women suffer worse healthcare outcomes in these examples, even when you control for socioeconomic status.

- To the extent that violence is either more permissible or more prevalent within certain communities, it can contribute to child abuse and domestic violence that leads to fractures, stabs, and gunshot wounds. Similarly, varying levels of police protection (and abuse) also represent social determinants of health. For example, if it is perceived within a community that law enforcement is less likely to patrol the area, the likelihood of violent crimes increases.[12]

Education, job opportunities, and income:

- Many components of socioeconomic status reflect subsequent health. A frequent consideration in patients subsequently having to present to emergency departments involves not being able to pay for routine medicines. In many instances, an otherwise controllable medical condition (e.g., asthma, seizures) exacerbates. Higher levels of education and income correlate with better health.[13]

Access to nutritious foods and physical activity opportunities:

- Food deserts describe communities with relatively limited access to nutrition and affordable food options. These communities are more likely to be present in urban and rural low-income neighborhoods that lack large supermarkets. A correlation exists between food deserts, the presence of obesity, and high incidences of diet-related diseases.[14] Similar considerations exist for communities with fewer parks and exercise facilities. Commercial physical activity facilities are less likely to be present in lower-income and racial minority neighborhoods. This finding, along with concerns regarding safety when engaging in outdoor physical activity, likely contributes to lower activity levels in these populations.[15]

Polluted air and water:

- Environmental toxins complicate our very existence. If the air we breathe and the water we drink negatively affect our health, we don't have as much of a chance to be healthy in the long run. Data show links between poor air and water quality, reduced socioeconomic status, and reduced health outcomes.[16]

Language and literacy skills:

- More commonly than one may think, language and literacy impact health. For many, the consideration is as simple as asking: how can someone follow instructions if they can't read or understand them? Accidental under- and overdosing on medications is a common occurrence and often results in suboptimal treatment or a new medical challenge from medication toxicity, respectively.

Just promoting healthy choices won't eliminate these and other health disparities. Instead, public health organizations and their partners in sectors like education, transportation, and housing need to take action to improve the conditions in people's environments. Those creating policy initiatives and those directly interacting with people need to consider the social environment. They must appreciate its impact, opportunities, and limitations that help or hinder the pursuit of health. Because the social circumstances and environment in which we live serve as major contributors to resulting healthcare disparities, any system or effort desiring to produce better healthcare outcomes would do well to start its efforts by analyzing the SDOH for those receiving care and allocating sufficient resources to address them.

CHAPTER TWO

THE STATUS QUO OF HEALTHCARE DELIVERY

I t's difficult to have a conversation about the American healthcare system because it can be hard to determine whether you're discussing the American healthcare system or the American healthcare industry, which aren't the same things. Similarly, a conversation about the general performance of the system isn't the same as discussing the wide variety in performance among different segments of the population within the system. This section highlights some of the important considerations of how healthcare services are delivered in America, reviews some important healthcare outcomes, challenges and opportunities, and leads to a proposed solution by the Managed Preventive Care Organization SIMPCO.

Most people are familiar with the work of Managed Care Organizations (MCO). Perhaps you're used to calling them something different, such as an HMO (Health Maintenance Organization), the first such entity (dating back to the early 1970s), a PPO (Preferred Provider Organization), or colloquially as "health insurance companies." Even more likely, you're familiar with some of them by name, such as Aetna/CVS

Health, Amerigroup, Anthem, BlueCross BlueShield, Centene/WellCare, Molina, and United Health Group.

Managed Care Organizations (MCOs) describe healthcare systems focused on reducing costs while maintaining quality of care. There are various tools used to accomplish this, such as the following:

- Contracting with groups of healthcare providers to establish rates on care and services (aka provider networks).
- Selecting specific primary care providers (PCPs) that one must see prior to having access to other specialists (at risk for otherwise not having services paid for).
- Needing prior authorization (approval) to get selected services, treatments, or medications.
- Using generic instead of branded medicines (aka prescription drug tiers).
- Engaging in selected preventive care efforts (e.g., check-ups, screenings, vaccinations).

MCOs have long been an attractive option for the federal and state governments administering Medicare and Medicaid because of the need to manage costs in addition to facilitating care. Regarding the contributions states have to make toward Medicaid, MCOs allow states to set and fix the amount of money they will pay on applicable healthcare services. It then becomes the responsibility of the MCOs –to their great risk and potentially great benefit– to manage those funds in enrolling eligible citizens and providing them with services. Of course, the inference is that the quality of care will not diminish as a result of MCOs' cost-control efforts via negotiations with hospitals, physicians and other participants in the healthcare system.

Unfortunately, the model often produces suboptimal results in producing systemic outcomes. Necessarily half of the states participating will be dissatisfied by performing below average compared to others. Inevitably, within every state, certain groups will perform less well than others. It particularly becomes problematic when the same demographic groups continually suffer worse outcomes on metrics of interest. These healthcare disparities are sometimes inherent in the model of the system, sometimes represent bias and discrimination (whether intended or not), and other times are adverse consequences related to the social determinants of health (SDOH).

What is the expected response in the latter set of examples? Are higher amounts of funds expected to be infused to attempt to eliminate adverse outcomes for selected subpopulations? Can these circumstances be addressed within the system with general programmatic efforts? Does the system as a whole decide to commit more dollars to preventive health and health promotion? These are parts of the ongoing challenges in perfecting a system of delivering care to hundreds of millions of citizens.

In spite of these challenges, American consumers (i.e., patients) generally express satisfaction with services received. In a national survey on experiences and satisfaction with healthcare, Medicaid enrollees gave their overall healthcare an average rating of 7.9 on a zero to ten scale. Forty-six percent gave their Medicaid coverage a score of nine or ten, while only 7.6% gave scores under five.[17] It's conceivable that patients may be oblivious to the overlying system of how MCOs works and don't personalize (or are even aware of) disparities produced by the system. It's possible that they use their specific experiences with their healthcare providers as a proxy as to whether the "system" functions well. However, as a dueling set of competing interests, the disconnect between patients' level of satisfaction and objective data on less ideal reflections of the system's performance doesn't prohibit the current system's continuation and growth.

Part of the challenge in improving the system of care delivery is the American healthcare system's reliance on Managed Care Organizations, which isn't just (or even primarily) a health or medical conversation. It's also an economic conversation. The data make the case explicitly.

- According to the Centers for Medicare & Medicaid Services, National Health Expenditures were $4.5 trillion in 2022 ($13,493 per person), representing 17.3% of Gross Domestic Product (GDP).[18] 2023 projections suggest a rise to $4.8 trillion.[19]
- Health care spending, both per person and as a share of GDP, continues to be far higher in the United States than in other high-income countries. Among the thirty-eight member countries of the Organization for Economic Co-operation and Development (OECD, existing to stimulate economic progress and world trade among most high-income, democratic nations committed to market economies), the US had the highest percentage of gross domestic product spent on health care in 2022. Switzerland, France, and Japan followed the US with dramatically smaller percentages, around 12% or lower.[18]

As an economic consideration, the US healthcare industry is a phenomenal success. It is the major driver of the US economy (followed by technology, construction, retail, and non-durable manufacturing).[20] With $4.5 trillion in revenue, healthcare profit pools reached $583 billion in 2022 and is expected to rise to $819 billion in 2027.[21] The healthcare industry added more than 650,000 jobs in 2023, growing at its fastest rate in more than three decades.[22,23]

It is this level of revenue generation, profitability, and job creation that supports the notion that moving from a market-based model of healthcare to a universal healthcare system would "wreck" the U.S. economy. Consider the following: in 2023, 91.2 million Americans were Medicaid recipients, representing coverage of healthcare services for the poor. Accordingly, in 2023, Medicare spending is estimated to have grown to over $1 trillion, and Medicaid spending is estimated at $852 billion. 2024 healthcare spending estimates per person is projected to rise to $15,074.[19] This level of cash infusion into the US economy sustains the economy. Its loss would create massive disruptions in commerce and employment if reduced in a meaningful manner.

However, a model that is meant to drive the economy and produce healthcare outcomes as a byproduct of doing so isn't as likely to produce optimal outcomes as a model that focuses on healthcare delivery, clinical excellence, and the pursuit of optimal outcomes. Particularly when considering the amount spent on healthcare in the US, the data leaves no other conclusion that this indeed has been the case. Consider the following data points from a comparison of high-income democratic nations committed to a market economy by The Commonwealth Fund. It is notable that the comparison concludes that the US produces the worst health outcomes overall of any high-income nation.[24]

- The US has the lowest life expectancy at birth.
- Americans are more likely to die younger.
- The US has the highest number of hospitalizations from preventable causes.
- The US has the highest death rates for avoidable or treatable conditions.

- The US has the highest maternal and infant mortality.
- The US has among the highest suicide rates.
- The US has the highest rate of people with multiple chronic conditions.
- The US has an obesity rate nearly twice the average.
- Americans see physicians less often than people in most other countries.
- The US has among the lowest rates of practicing physicians and hospital beds per 1,000 population.

One of the foremost challenges is, in its emphasis on the economics of healthcare (and perhaps in support of citizens' desire to freely live their lives as they see fit), the US appears firmly committed to a curative-care (aka "sick care") model of medicine over a system of health prevention and health promotion. The American healthcare system's efforts too often involve identifying disease (and thus identifying opportunities for high revenue-generating use of technology, surgeries, and other processes and procedures) more than sustaining health. As such, whereas our screening rates for cancers are among the highest for comparable nations, our vaccination rates fall behind. Our use of expensive technologies, including CT scans and MRIs, is higher than that of our peer group of nations. Our use of specialized procedures, such as hip replacement surgery, is higher. This approach works very well in stimulating the healthcare sector and the overall economy but not as well in producing a healthy society.

Attempts to objectify performance by international entities that rank the national healthcare system have produced the following results.

- In terms of overall efficiency, the World Health Organization (WHO) ranks the US healthcare system 47th.[25]

- US News and World Report ranks the US healthcare system 23rd.[26]
- CEOWORLD Magazine ranks the US healthcare system 15th.[27]
- The Legatum Prosperity Index for 2023 ranks the US healthcare system 69th.[28]

Further evidence of the United States' commitment to curative care in its health model and its relatively insufficient support of health prevention and promotion is found in two simple and telling statistics.

- Nearly forty percent of all deaths in the United States are due to behavioral causes, including tobacco use, consuming an unhealthy diet, physical inactivity, and excessive drinking, meaning citizens have control of foreseeable and preventable causes of death.[29]
- The US spends less than three percent of its spending on public health and prevention.[30]

Reconciling the amount of money spent in the US healthcare system with optimal outcomes is an ongoing challenge. Fortunately, the path to doing so has always been clearly described in public health research.

CHAPTER THREE

DEFINING THE OUNCE OF PREVENTION

It has been a given around the world's healthcare systems that "an ounce of prevention is worth a pound of cure." However, what isn't as appreciated is that preventive healthcare involves distinct components of primary, secondary, and tertiary prevention.

Primary prevention is reducing the occurrence of disease by avoiding and controlling modifiable risk factors. A typical example involves avoiding cigarette smoke and smoking as a means of reducing the risk of lung cancer. Secondary prevention is the early detection of disease prior to development of clinical signs and symptoms. This occurs commonly with screening examinations (e.g., for breast and prostate cancer). Tertiary prevention is the control of already-developed disease as a means of preventing additional, and typically worse, complications.

Whether primary, secondary, or tertiary preventive efforts are offered, it's important to engage these efforts based on whether services are occurring in clinical/medical settings versus in community/population-based settings. Here are some examples of how this typically can be done.

Clinical Prevention:

- Primary preventive efforts include the administration of immunizations and lifestyle (behavioral) counseling on matters such as diet, exercise, or stress avoidance.
- Secondary preventive efforts include testing for early detection of common causes of death (e.g., cancer, heart disease).
- Tertiary preventive efforts include disease management and care of chronic illnesses in the most proactive ways still available, depending on a patient's condition.

Community/Population-Based Prevention:

- Primary preventive efforts include attempts to transform the mindset of communities and otherwise address the social determinants of health by improving conditions within a community environment. Common examples include the administration of health information fairs, community and work-based wellness programs, having access to reliable information via the internet, media, other means of information technology that provides self-assessment tools, and passage of legislation. Notable past examples of legislation that represents primary prevention include laws requiring seat belts, motorcycle helmets, and indoor smoking bans.
- Secondary preventive efforts include health fairs that feature testing and disease screening.
- Tertiary preventive efforts include disease management outside of the clinical setting, including

home health care, school initiatives, and work (occupational) health initiatives.

Understanding the differences in these levels of prevention has become much more important in modern times. Healthcare systems and institutions have tended to focus more on secondary and tertiary prevention. It's relevant to note that in addition to the patient health benefit, emphasis on these efforts in the clinical setting also creates economic benefit when subsequent surgeries and other medical evaluations and procedures are needed.

However, as people have become more inclined to become self-informed on matters of health and disease, traditional exclusive reliance on and trust in healthcare institutions has lessened. Some of this involves informed self-determination, but in a significant number of examples, misinformation, disinformation, politicization of medical science, and a lack of clear, transparent, and accessible information from within their healthcare settings have eroded the public trust.[31] This evolution highlights the need to redouble efforts toward giving people primary prevention and community-based prevention and to have accurate information from trusted messengers get through to them.

This is a good place to point out that in the US healthcare system, only three percent of the money spent goes towards these types of public health and preventive efforts, including government-funded and private industry efforts.[32]

CHAPTER FOUR

EFFICIENCIES IN HEALTHCARE: EFFECTIVE PREVENTIVE HEALTH AND BENDING THE COST CURVE

Public health data supports the contention that an ounce of prevention (i.e., preventive care) is worth a pound of cure (i.e., curative care). Of course, you'd intuitively believe this in the same way you could hardly eat enough fruits and vegetables to approximate the cost of any obesity-related surgeries, and it's important to know that you'd still be healthier with the preventive efforts than from receiving the surgery. Still, it's important to be able to quantify cause and effect. The American and Canadian Public Health Associations (APHA and CPHA) have compiled data on various public health initiatives and published the following analyses of return on investment (ROI) on them, ranked from highest to lowest.[33]

Intervention	ROI
Child safety seat	3900%
Water fluoridation	3700%
Mental health and addiction	3600%
Tobacco prevention	1900%
Vaccination	1500%
Early education	1300%
Biking and walking opportunities	1200%
Food and nutrition	1000%
Childhood health and development	800%
Workplace safety	500%
Cleaner vehicles	300%
Tobacco cessation	125%

Additional research also shows positive ROI on different types of public health initiatives.

- A notable seven-year study involving over 10,000 people in a workplace environment showed a return on investment estimated to be $2.53 for every dollar spent on health promotion.[34]
- A study in the Harvard Business Review showed an ROI on comprehensive, well-run employee wellness programs could be as high as 6 to 1.[35]
- An analysis at the University of Chicago showed an ROI for every $1 invested in targeted mental health actions brings a return of $4 in benefits realized through decreased absenteeism, improved productivity, and reductions in workers' compensation claims.[36]
- The Trust for America's Health estimates that community-based interventions could save $5.60 for every $1 invested.[37]

The National Institutes of Health estimates delivery of primary preventive services to 90% of the population could reduce expenditures by $53.9 billion (3.1% of 2006 personal healthcare expenditures) at a cost of $52.1 billion, representing a net cost reduction of $1.8 billion (0.1% of 2006 personal healthcare expenditures). The closer you get to identifying a disease that requires medical treatment (via secondary and tertiary preventive services), the more cost reductions become lower.[38]

If and as goals exist to bend the cost curve and to empower individuals to become more responsible for their health, it is critical that efforts to expand primary prevention and community-based preventive efforts are made.

Given the demonstrated high return on investment by preventive health measures, investing in health prevention and promotion should be prioritized. The notion that costs can be simply cut, and the industry would simply accommodate without consequences, is flawed and would cost lives. Therefore, conversations on bending the cost curve are better thought of as achieving greater value from healthcare spend than just finding ways to cut costs. Redistributing healthcare spending based on higher value relative to the resource investment will produce incremental and overall higher economic savings and better healthcare outcomes.

What does this involve practically? As an example, based on the better return on investment for primary preventive health efforts, they should be prioritized over secondary and tertiary preventive efforts. It is important to note that this point is an affirmation of primary prevention and not a repudiation of secondary and tertiary prevention.

When seeking to reduce costs or services, the same consideration of value is important. Costly services that incrementally and/or objectively show less benefit to patient outcomes should be prioritized less and be accompanied by a proportionately lower resource investment. This premise underlies the Managed Care Organizations' practice of prior authorization.

This premise of focusing on obtaining higher value from healthcare spend has been objectified, and preventive services that offer high value in this way have been clearly identified. The U.S. Preventive Services Task Force has identified a core set of clinical preventive services with established effectiveness. Of twenty-five such services reviewed by the National Commission on Prevention Priorities, fifteen cost less than $35,000 per quality-adjusted life year produced (QALY, meaning one year in perfect health).[38]

Cost-Effectiveness of 15 Out of 25 Clinical Preventive Services Reviewed by the National Commission on Prevention Priorities

Cost-effectiveness (CE) ratio < 0 (cost saving)	Preventive Service. Advising at-risk adults to take aspirin. Childhood immunization. Smoking cessation advice and help to quit. Screening adults for alcohol misuse and brief counseling. Vision screening (for adults aged 65 and older).
CE ratio = $0–13,999/QALY	Chlamydia screening (sexually active adolescents and young women). Colorectal cancer screening (adults aged 50 and older). Influenza immunization (adults aged 50 and older). Pneumococcal immunization (adults aged 65 and older). Vision screening in preschool-age children.
CE ratio = $14,000–34,999/QALY	Cervical cancer screening (all women). Counseling women of childbearing age to take folic acid supplements. Counseling women to use calcium supplements. Injury prevention counseling for parents of young children. Hypertension screening (all adults).

The Community Task Force on Preventive Services has identified a similar cadre of effective population-based interventions.[39]

Clinical Preventive Service	Type of Prevention	Description and Target Population
Tetanus-diphtheria booster	Primary	Immunize adults every 10 years.
Folic acid use	Primary	Counsel women of childbearing age routinely on the use of folic acid supplements to prevent birth defects.
Chlamydia screening	Primary	Screen sexually active women under age 25 routinely.
Pneumococcal immunization	Primary	Immunize adults aged 65 and older against pneumococcal disease with one dose.
Osteoporosis screening	Primary	Screen routinely women aged 65 and older and age 60 and older at increased risk for osteoporosis and discuss the benefits and harms of treatment options
Influenza immunization	Primary	Immunize adults aged 50 and older against influenza once annually.
Obesity screening	Primary	Screen adults aged 18 and older routinely for obesity and offer high-intensity counseling about diet, exercise, or both, together with behavioral interventions for at least 1 year.
Cholesterol screening	Primary	Screen routinely for lipid disorders among men aged 35 and older and women aged 45 and older and treat with lipid-lowering drugs to prevent cardiovascular disease.
Alcohol screening	Primary	Screen adults aged 18 and older routinely to identify those whose alcohol

Clinical Preventive Service	Type of Prevention	Description and Target Population
		use places them at increased risk and provide brief counseling with follow-up.
Tobacco	Primary	Screen adults aged 18 and older for tobacco use, provide brief counseling, offer medication, and make referrals for more intensive counseling.
Hypertension screening	Primary	Measure blood pressure routinely in all adults aged 18 and older and treat with antihypertensive medication to prevent cardiovascular disease.
Childhood immunizations	Primary	Immunize children under age 5 against diphtheria, tetanus, pertussis, measles, mumps, rubella, polio, *Haemophilus influenza* type b, varicella, pneumococcal, and influenza.
Daily aspirin use	Primary	Discuss daily aspirin use with men aged 40 and older, women aged 50 and older, and others at increased risk to prevent heart disease.
Depression screening	Secondary	Screen adults aged 18 and older for depression in clinical practices with systems in place to assure accurate diagnosis, treatment and follow-up.
Hearing screening	Secondary	Screen for hearing impairments in adults aged 65 and older and make referrals to specialists for treatment.
Breast cancer screening	Secondary	Screen women aged 50 and older routinely with mammography alone or with clinical breast examination and discuss screening with women 40–49 to choose an age to initiate screening.
Vision screening	Cross-classified	Screen children under age 5 routinely to detect amblyopia, strabismus, and defects in visual acuity.
Vision screening	Cross-classified	Screen adults aged 65 and older routinely for diminished vision with the Snellen visual acuity chart and make referrals.

Clinical Preventive Service	Type of Prevention	Description and Target Population
Cervical cancer screening	Cross-classified	Screen women who have been sexually active and have a cervix within 3 years of onset of sexual activity or age 21 routinely with cervical cytology (Pap smears).
Colorectal cancer screening	Cross-classified	Screen adults aged 50 and older routinely with fecal occult blood test, sigmoidoscopy, or colonoscopy.

Prioritizing the above initiatives as part of the delivery of health and medical care is a means test that improves quality and optimizes costs.

The healthcare industry is a major part of the American economy and needs to be monitored in ways that ensure healthy growth and financial contributions back into society. The healthcare system may not have established that universal health is a right in America, but America's financial commitment to health far exceeds any other nation's investment. To that end, ongoing efforts to apply outcomes-based and evidence-based efforts to improve society health should be under continual scrutiny as well.

The Institute of Medicine (US) Roundtable on Evidence-Based Medicine offers the following algorithm as a way to test healthcare efforts and contribute toward bending the cost curve and focusing on high-value initiatives.[38]

• Does the intervention improve health outcomes, and how strong is the evidence?

• If the intervention is effective, is it cost-effective (a good value)?

• Can other options achieve better results or the same results at a lower cost?

The healthcare quality and cost-effective conversations are

not mutually exclusive. We should be at least as concerned with the relatively poor healthcare outcomes as we are with the level of healthcare spending. Proceeding in this manner can address both concerns.

CHAPTER FIVE

THE STERLING INITIATIVES MANAGED PREVENTIVE CARE ORGANIZATION (SIMPCO): THE PRACTICE OF PREVENTIVE HEALTH

In the United States, we assume that public health initiatives should both improve outcomes and save money. Other countries that invest a high percentage of their healthcare spend into health prevention and promotion do so because they realize that prevention might not produce immediate cost savings, but those investments are often massively cost-effective in the long run. These efforts include vaccination programs, antismoking campaigns, and interventions like bolstering sanitation and promoting clean water access. Price Waterhouse Coopers estimates that the US could save almost $500 billion per year by addressing obesity, smoking, and other modifiable risk factors.[40]

To be fair, there are a plethora of preventive health organizations in America, many of whom offer components of public health best practices to great success. However, what hasn't been brought to fruition is a full commitment to the clinical practice of preventive health. Public health has been expressed more as a series of policy proclamations to be incorporated into the prevailing health and medical care system than a constellation of individual best practices to be engaged and delivered in a comprehensive manner. Preventive health requires focused implementation. The practice of preventive health has yet to become a part of the American health industry's landscape.

INTRODUCTION

Improving the health of Americans who cannot afford to pay for healthcare has been Medicaid's primary goal since 1965. Medicaid has been stretched and revamped in many different ways through the years, often due to out-of-control costs associated with medical care. However, the goals have remained the same.

Our unique place in history, the era immediately after the implementation of the Affordable Care Act (ACA) and Medicaid expansion, heralds large Managed Care Organizations (MCO) as the newest sculptors of America's healthcare landscape. These MCOs now accept over a trillion federal dollars annually toward delivering improved quality of care and greater access to care. They have drastically reduced costs and the rate of rise of costs to State and Federal Medicaid budgets.

Over ten years after the implementation of this grand effort, a new opportunity is apparent. While there are many routes various MCOs have pursued to achieve these outcomes, certain challenges have remained. These challenges include providing roughly equal access to all communities, offering health prevention and embracing newer technologies. These concerns are present across America. Fortunately, improvements in public health strategy in implementing the aims and challenges of health provision now exist and represent best practices awaiting implementation. To this end, in 2019, we created America's first "Managed Preventive Care Organization (MPCO)," an entity to be known as SIMPCO.

The Sterling Initiatives Managed Preventive Care

Organization (SIMPCO) concept was proposed to be a new, common-sense paradigm for improving the health of Americans. At its core are the types of preventive health services available to a smaller than optimal percentage of the MCOs' Medicaid demographic, though they are often more readily available to privately insured clients. SIMPCO means MPCOs will take place alongside the MCOs and focus on complementary services that enhance the collective efforts of the MCOs. The efforts of MPCOs would produce specific outcomes, including increasing access to care and improving both objective and perceived quality of healthcare services in its markets.

These initiatives have been individually demonstrated to be effective not only in improving members' health but also in ensuring appropriate utilization of care. The focus on prevention and aligning resources with appropriate portals of entry into the healthcare system have been shown to lead to dramatic long-term savings. This occurs in several specific ways. First, these efforts expend a mere fraction of the current costs of medical care. Secondly, these efforts reduce avoidable visits to emergency departments, which represent the most expensive portals of entry into the healthcare system (not to mention that in 2021, there were over 140 million total emergency department visits in the US[41]). Additionally, preventive measures forestall the development of chronic disease, surgeries, and other medical endeavors that expend tremendous resources with diminishing returns in too many instances.

In her January 16, 2014, memo, "Reducing Nonurgent Use of Emergency Departments and Improving Appropriate Care in Appropriate Settings," Cindy Mann, Director of the Centers for Medicare and Medicaid, opens with this statement.[42]

The Centers for Medicare & Medicaid Services (CMS) has been strengthening our collaborations with states in order to reduce costs, improve the patient experience, and improve the health of the populations we serve. As beneficiaries gain coverage as a result of the Affordable Care Act, utilization of services across the healthcare system is likely to increase, and *states and CMS share a strong interest in reducing unnecessary hospital emergency department (ED) usage. In this changing environment, CMS is committed to partnering with states, plans, providers, and consumers to implement reforms that can appropriately address the needs of our beneficiaries more effectively and efficiently.* [author's emphasis]

By definition, the Managed Preventive Care Organization concept aligns with Director Mann's astute leadership. SIMPCO seeks to accomplish these goals with our focus on providing greater access to care, modernizing healthcare delivery, and educating members about medically proven risk reduction and primary, secondary, and tertiary disease prevention techniques in a way that empowers individuals to become better stewards of their own healthcare and communities to rally around health prevention and promotion.

Three primary factors have been identified that lead to inappropriate use of Emergency Department resources: fear, lack of knowledge and lack of access to alternative means of care. Due to the infusion of approximately 30 million new U.S. citizens into the healthcare system via the Affordable Care Act and Medicaid, these problems are being exacerbated by straining resources in the midst of a national shortage of physicians (projected as being up to 86,000 less than needed by 2036 by the Association of American Medical Colleges).[43]

Furthermore, the resultant over-utilization of emergency rooms jeopardizes quality with its resource utilization, all the while caring for a large patient load, which can be seen in fewer costs and less labor-intensive aspects of the spectrum of care.[44] It is also notable that community-driven initiatives have not been sufficiently prominent in developing culturally sensitive and specific approaches to care. This leaves one of every five eligible beneficiaries still without options beyond utilizing more expensive portals of entry into the healthcare system, most notably the local emergency room. The demographics of these eligible beneficiaries meet the capabilities of the MPCO to close the gap further and uniquely.

SIMPCO is a free enterprise innovation. It is a physician-led, public health-driven, Minority Business Enterprise offering that delivers many desired solutions to complement the work of Managed Care Organizations, corporations, governmental agencies and other stakeholders. The most cogent of these solutions includes improving access to established methods of traditional care, providing means for enhanced preventive care and offering remedies for inappropriately high levels of healthcare resource utilization. The roster of SIMPCO services supplements and relieves the burden on both primary and emergency care systems.

Within SIMPCO, we consolidate and coordinate the following healthcare best practices.

- Use of navigators for enrollment into Managed Care Organizations (MCOs)
- Use of Administrative Personal Healthcare Consultants (APHCs) for home health maintenance between medical office visits
- Use of Clinical Personal Healthcare Consultants (CPHCs) for telehealth (health information and advice)
- Use of telehealth to provide episodic information and advice to enrollees, including mental telehealth
- Use of call centers to interact with MCOs and facilitate telehealth and telemedicine offerings
- Care coordination to facilitate utilization of the full spectrum of eligible health services, including

enrollment in and reporting to MCOs and engagement of MCOs for delivery of clinical secondary and tertiary preventive services (e.g., screenings and testing)
- Combining community engagement and empowerment with data analysis to drive interest and participation in one's health

MEETING THE CHALLENGE OF CMS

As noted by former Director of CMS Cindy Mann, CMS challenges can be best met via a three-tiered strategy which involves: (1) broadening access to primary care services; (2) focusing on frequent ED users, i.e., "super-utilizers" and (3) targeting the needs of people with behavioral health problems. This approach is deemed most effective for improving patient experience and public health at a lower cost. Managed Preventive Care Organization (MPCO) developed by SIMPCO offers solutions in line with this strategy, as outlined below.

1. Broaden access to primary care services

Primary care services begin with access to professional medical information and advice presented via easily accessible and easily understood modalities. SIMPCO will not only broaden access to MCOs via its navigator enrollment strategies but will also provide preventive services via our telehealth and telemedicine components. As education and reliable information is the key to disease prevention, our clients—even those in rural and underprivileged communities—can gain timely access to these services in several formats using a personal computer or a smartphone. This is a viable strategy given that, according to the 2023 Pew Research Regarding Cell Phones[45]:

- 95% of US adults use the internet

- 90% of US adults have a smartphone
- 80% of US adults subscribe to high-speed internet at home

SIMPCO also provides direct access to experts, thereby reducing the burden on the emergency departments (EDs) or forcing patients to wait for weeks for appointments with primary care providers. As members can now receive immediate information and advice about pressing medical concerns, they are empowered to make good health choices for themselves and their families while ensuring that vital emergency systems of care are available to those who truly need them.

2. Focus on frequent ED users – "super-utilizers"

By introducing Personal Healthcare Consultants (PHCs) to the American healthcare landscape, our primary objective is to shift the "super-utilizers" to the SIMPCO suite of services where they can access all relevant, high-quality information and advice. Our PHCs are trained to identify ED "super-utilizers," and their aim is to directly engage them in our dynamic, interactive education and advice services. By adopting this proactive strategy, we believe that we can resolve the underlying issues and encourage them to comply with best health practices, thereby decreasing inappropriate ED utilization. By giving these individuals access to telehealth and telemedicine services and expediting return visits to their MCOs, PHCs will serve as the MPCO equivalent of case managers in the MCO model. In this regard, the SIMPCO core objectives are: (1) promoting a "virtual preventive medical home," (2) coordinating care among providers, and (3) maintaining client engagement in preventive care activities.

3. Target the needs of people with behavioral health problems

Several of our PHCs are behavioral health experts who are

available 24/7—by telephone (via telehealth) and online—to direct patients with mental health and substance abuse issues to the appropriate services. SIMPCO also will coordinate and facilitate care needs with MCOs in real-time.

The SIMPCO model of managed preventive care and education addresses the opportunity for producing better healthcare outcomes, bending the healthcare cost curve and optimizing financial resources. It seeks to transform communities by elevating the importance of health prevention and promotion within them and their residents. This is done in a person-centric, culturally sensitive manner, bringing the best practices of public health to bear toward addressing social determinants of health and combating healthcare disparities. These efforts will be followed by ongoing public health research tailored to the unique environments of each community we serve.

These efforts are to be administered in health and human service facilities (aka "Health Hubs") to populations now able and willing to become better stewards of their own health while coordinating services with other components of the healthcare system. SIMPCO's health hubs will provide spaces for health education activities covering wellness, nutrition and diet, activity and exercise, mental health, and disease management. SIMPCO's campuses will include sufficient, safe green spaces for community gathering and activity. Our facilities include offices for quarterly health checkups. Our mobile health hub includes provisions for mental and physician telehealth.

SIMPCO's use of public health best practices and coordinating these efforts under one room within communities with strategy partners is the practice of preventive health. This is the SIMPCO Solution.

CHAPTER SIX

THE ILLINOIS EXAMPLE

The State of Illinois was an ideal location to pursue the implementation of the Managed Preventive Care Organization. Illinois has an ongoing history of proactively assessing the healthcare needs of its citizens, allocating resources to respond to those needs, and adjusting as needed. In the last fifteen years alone, Illinois has taken several steps to be innovative and in alignment with best practices. Some of those efforts have included the following:

- Illinois began the transition to Medicaid-managed care in 2011, starting with thirty counties. By January 2018, it launched HealthChoice Illinois, expanding to all 102 of its counties. As of May 2024, about 2.73 million of Illinois' 3.48 million Medicaid members are now enrolled in managed care.[46]
- On February 22, 2013, the Department of Health and Human Services announced that the State of Illinois would partner with the Centers for Medicare & Medicaid Services (CMS) to test a new model for providing Medicare-Medicaid enrollees with a more

coordinated, person-centered care experience. Under the demonstration, called the Medicare-Medicaid Alignment Initiative (MMAI), Illinois and CMS began contracting with health plans to coordinate the delivery of and be accountable for all covered Medicare and Medicaid services for participating enrollees.

- Illinois opted to expand Medicaid eligibility, as allowed by the Affordable Care Act, in July 2013 (for a January 1, 2014, effective date), making Medicaid available to an increased number of low-income, non-elderly adults.
- The Illinois Department of Healthcare and Family Services launched the Healthcare Transformation Collaboratives in 2021. The ongoing program aims to close gaps in healthcare services and eliminate barriers to access and inequities that persist in Illinois' healthcare system. The stated goal of Healthcare Transformation Collaboratives is to reorient the healthcare delivery system in Illinois around people and communities. The Transformation Plan contains four major components:
- Community Needs (Focus on community needs for all levels of healthcare with an emphasis on addressing social and structural determinants of health)
- Health and Wellness (Improve health and wellness for individuals and communities)
- Specialized Approaches (Tailor solutions to meet the unique needs of individuals) and
- Sustainable Investments (Invest in projects, large and small, that improve outcomes, decrease disparities, and are sustainable over time)

These various efforts address the challenges of Illinois' health system from multiple angles.

In doing the above, Illinois' financial commitment to healthcare is substantial. In Governor J.B. Pritzker's proposed fiscal year 2025 (FY25) budget, funds to the state's Department of Healthcare and Family Services totaled almost $39.5 billion, with a projected Medicaid liability of $26.8 billion. As proposed, healthcare expenditures represented 32% of the budget and were the largest line item in state government.[47]

With respect to outcomes, the Illinois example is not dissimilar to what occurs on the federal level. Illinois, despite a large and ongoing financial commitment to healthcare, remains among the middle tier of states with respect to healthcare outcomes. Illinois also confronts significant disparities between its various diverse populations, including adverse outcomes for certain racial ethnicities and rural populations relative to urban geographic locations.

These disparities manifested in the worst possible way during the COVID-19 pandemic. Illinois (and Chicago specifically) experienced a level of mortality in certain populations that brought into full view how social determinants of health and healthcare disparities impact the expression of disease.

- A review of the top 10 zip codes in Chicago suffering deaths during the COVID-19 pandemic showed residents of predominantly Black and Latinx populations suffered almost three times the number of mortalities as did those in the top ten suffering White communities.[1]
- The adverse outcomes experienced were not only based on lack of access to medical care but were dramatically impacted by the baseline health status of residents within certain zip codes. Factors in these zip

codes included distinguishing social considerations, including a lack of available personal protective equipment (PPE), the existence of medical deserts, and crowded home environments more likely to promote contagion than home environments in other communities.

- Ironically and to their detriment, these communities also expressed higher skepticism of the dangers of the disease and the efficacy of immunizations. In part, this reflected a relative paucity of trusted messengers to sort through valid information, disinformation, and misinformation.

I came to this conversation keen on a proposal that had been decades in the making. Having been born and having later completed my emergency medicine residency at Chicago's Cook County Hospital (now the John Stroger Hospital of Cook County), I was a direct product of the state's hospital. I was a recipient of its care and professionally inclined to address the care of communities based on my training there. Those considerations were enhanced by my experiences during medical school when I had an opportunity to combine my medical training at the University of Illinois College of Medicine with a public health and business degree from Harvard University's T.C. Chan School of Public Health (HSPH).

At Harvard, my concentration was in Health Policy and Management, meaning I got training in both the business and policy sides of health care. Being at Harvard meant I had access to amazing thought and industry leaders in both areas throughout its schools of public health, business, and government. One such individual was William Hsiao, who famously developed the resource-based relative value scale (RBRVS) by which physician fees for seeing patients are determined. In doing so, "relative value" in resources expended was assigned to different physician services, actions, and specialties. He had been named Man of the Year in Medicine in 1989, just as I came to HSPH. Hsiao was my mentor while I was at Harvard and ended up being my principal sponsor on one of my two biggest projects while there: the conceptualization of a health and human services center as a vehicle for providing healthcare.

Through my personal experiences and during my training, it was obvious that medical care (aka curative care, aka "sick care") wasn't sufficient to address the needs of keeping people healthy. I knew the real-world needs of having to choose between having to pay for a family meal versus getting a prescription filled. I understood that levels of illiteracy and language barriers effectively prohibited some people from following the instructions necessary to follow treatment regimens. I grew up in a place where your zip code and accompanying considerations within your neighborhood had a greater impact on your life expectancy than the natural order would have otherwise chosen. Here's a case in point: my father died from a stray gunshot when I was six years old while simply walking down the street.

The idea of the health and human services center was to assemble professionals within a community space to help people achieve health – but not solely through the delivery of medicine. The Health and Human Services Center is meant to find ways to clear the barriers people have while pursuing health. As proposed, it included offering job training, educational activities (e.g., obtaining GEDs), resources to provide jobs, and financial credentialing for medical services. The center was to be a community gathering place while all these activities - and many more – occurred under one roof.

Another thing I learned about public health was within America, the idea of "the practice of preventive health" wasn't yet part of the healthcare landscape. There has been a stubborn and incorrect conflation of healthcare and medical care. The current system design has held on to the notion that the best practices of public health were to be contained within the practice of medicine. Of course, there have been multiple entities that separately address various components of health prevention and promotion (e.g., wellness programs and screening facilities) but not in a comprehensive way analogous to how physicians care for patients.

In real-time, professionally, I had no way of knowing that the practice of emergency medicine would bring to light many of the exact failings of the medical care system that my proposed health and human services center was meant to address. Whether by design or happenstance, emergency departments have become the safety nets for the American healthcare system. Emergency medicine is the largest component of the medical system, and it addresses the care of those without insurance or a medical home with a family physician or other provider.

Unfortunately, and as a practical matter, that's alarmingly inefficient on multiple fronts. Emergency departments are the most expensive portals of entry into the healthcare system, with costs that are up to twenty-two times more than those of a visit to a primary care facility and even more than the cost of using telehealth or telemedicine.[48] Systemic reviews of emergency department visits estimate that approximately thirty-two percent of patients presenting to emergency rooms could have been seen in a primary care setting.[49] The combination of these last two principles reveals billions of avoidable costs to the healthcare system and is a major contributor to the ongoing financial failures of hospitals across the country. In fact, an analysis of nearly twenty-four million emergency department visits across 750 hospitals projected an estimated $8.3 billion in annual savings could be had if that same care had been provided in another treatment setting.[50]

On the clinical side, little about being seen in an emergency department represents the promotion of health. Far too often, patients are seen and returned to the same conditions that produced their pathology. Emergency departments can be viewed as the final common meeting place for the adverse consequences of the social determinants of health. The best we often can do to promote health in emergency departments is to take advantage of the patient's shock while in a moment of crisis and hope to convince them to make definitive changes to their lifestyles. In addition, and when we're lucky, the opportunity presents to refer patients to a primary care physician or other provider for ongoing care. In many community settings, the latter consideration happens a lot less frequently than you may be inclined to believe. One 2016 study in the Annals of Emergency Medicine shows that only 30.7% of patients were able to get an appointment within seven days of their emergency room visit; the success rate was even worse for Medicaid patients (25.5%).[51]

Then came COVID. The pandemic simply exposed the reality that better healthcare outcomes aren't optimally produced by focusing on creating better medical facilities but by creating better health and ensuring better access to healthcare. When the crisis hit and the data exposed death rates that were wildly different based on demographics, it became time to act. There has not been a complete demonstration that inadequate attention and emphasis on prevention creates foreseeable and preventable human and economic crises due to disease. The prevention imperative became understood.

After approximately ten years of advocating for the effort in Illinois, In 2022, the Illinois General Assembly passed a demonstration project for a Managed Preventive Care and Education Organization for fiscal years 2023-2027 at an amount of $60 million annually for five years. In 2024, the Illinois Department of Healthcare and Family Services released a Request for Applications to establish Managed Preventive Care and Education Organizations (MPCEOs) across the State.

SIMPCO is proud to have successfully advocated for the establishment of the practice of preventive health in Illinois. We will continue to seek to expand this effort on the federal level and within additional states across America. We look forward to compiling and reporting data that results from these efforts.

CHAPTER SEVEN

TRANSFORMING AMERICA INTO A CULTURE OF HEALTH

It can be said that one's good health is a result of thousands of correct decisions. Ultimately, these decisions are best facilitated by an infrastructure in which people can participate that provides the opportunity for them to stay healthy instead of attempting to get well. As previously discussed, the differences between primary, secondary, and tertiary preventive care are the differences between using knowledge to maintain health, testing to prevent and starve off disease, and efforts to avoid the worst consequences of disease that have emerged.

The American healthcare system drives the American economy. The uniquely American healthcare system can be maintained and embraced while enhancing health prevention and promotion through efforts such as SIMPCO's managed preventive care organization. Policymakers should take solace in (and, in fact, be excited by) the knowledge that investments in health prevention and promotion bring a significant return on investment. Such efforts are not only good for business but good for the economy. The SIMPCO model isn't necessarily in competition with the managed care organization (MCO) model; it should be viewed as complementary. Coordination of care in ways that bend the cost curve, grow the economy, and produce better health and healthcare outcomes for the population is exactly what the system means to offer.

America has long been the most productive nation on earth. Most of that productivity stems from labor forces that are healthy enough to work. Work doesn't have to take a toll on one's health. Workplaces, schools, and other components of society are made better and more productive when society embraces and prioritizes health. America's economic advantages could still be greater by developing a culture of health.

It bears noting that the times require solutions that involve individuals taking a larger role in their healthcare. An annual physical with intermittent emergency department visits was never a comprehensive enough approach to health. In the American healthcare system, there is room for both the practice of medicine and the practice of preventive health. The ongoing escalation of costs for an approach dominated by curative care considerations to the detriment of preventive care is not sustainable. The time is now to embrace health prevention and promotion with a dedicated focus. We offer the Managed Preventive Care Organization.

ENDNOTES

1. Blaser, M. et al. COVID-19 Mortality in Chicagoland: Data Limitations and Solutions. https://publichealth. uic.edu/news-stories/covid-19-mortality-in- chicagoland-data-limitations-and-solutions/ Accessed July 11, 2024.

2. Annie FH, Crews C, Drabish K, Mandapaka S. Effect of Coal Mining on Health Outcomes Between Male and Female Miners in Southern West Virginia: A Brief Report. Cureus. 2023 Nov 18;15(11):e49009. doi: 10.7759/cureus.49009. PMID: 38111417; PMCID: PMC10726975.

3. Harrison Wein, Ph.D. Health in Rural America: Connecting to Care. National Institutes of Health, March 2022, https://newsinhealth.nih.- gov/2022/03/health-rural-america#

4. Devna Bose, Mississippi Ranks as the Unhealthiest State in the Entire Country, Again. June 22, 2023. https://mississippitoday.org/2023/06/22/ mississippi-health-rankings-worst-in-country/

5. Healthy People 2030, U.S. Department of Health and Human Services, Office of Disease Prevention and Health Promotion. Retrieved from https://health.gov/healthypeople/objectives-and-data/social-determinants-health

6. Arias E, Xu JQ, Kochanek KD. United States life tables, 2021. National Vital Statistics Reports; vol 72 no 12. Hyattsville, MD: National Center for Health Statistics. 2023. DOI: https://dx.doi.org/10.15620/cdc:132418.

7. National Vital Statistics System mortality data, 2010-2022.

8. U.S. Centers for Disease Control and Prevention. Leading Causes of Death in Rural America Partner Toolkit. Accessed at https://www.cdc.gov/rural-health/php/causes-of-death/index.html#:~:text=CDC%20da-ta%20show%20that%20peo-ple,of%20these%20deaths%20are%20preventable.

9. Hoffman KM, Trawalter S, Axt JR, Oliver MN. Racial bias in pain assessment and treatment recommendations, and false beliefs about biological differences between blacks and whites. Proc Natl Acad Sci U S A. 2016 Apr 19;113(16):4296-301. doi: 10.1073/pnas.1516047113. Epub 2016 Apr 4. PMID: 27044069; PMCID: PMC4843483.

10. CDC 2022. Infant mortality in the United States, 2020: Data from the period

11. linked birth/infant death file. National Vital Statistics Reports. Table 2.

12. https://stacks.cdc.gov/view/cdc/120700

13. Hoyert DL. Maternal mortality rates in the United States, 2021. NCHS Health E-Stats. 2023. DOI: https://dx.doi.org/10.15620/cdc:124678

14. Ratcliffe, J.H. et al. (2011). The Philadelphia foot patrol experiment: A randomized controlled trial of police patrol effectiveness in violent crime hotspots. *Criminology, 49(3)*, 795-831.

15. Zajacova A, Lawrence EM. The Relationship Between Education and Health: Reducing Disparities Through a Contextual Approach. Annu Rev Public Health. 2018 Apr 1;39:273-289. doi: 10.1146/annurev-publhealth-031816-044628. Epub 2018 Jan 12. PMID: 29328865; PMCID: PMC5880718.

16. National Research Council (US). The Public Health Effects of Food Deserts: Workshop Summary. Washington (DC): National Academies Press (US); 2009. Summary. Available from: https://www.ncbi.nlm.nih.gov/books/NBK208018/

17. Powell LM, Slater S, Chaloupka FJ, Harper D. Availability of physical activity-related facilities and neighborhood demographic and socioeconomic characteristics: a national study. Am J Public Health. 2006 Sep;96(9):1676-80. doi: 10.2105/AJPH.2005.065573. Epub 2006 Jul 27. PMID: 16873753; PMCID: PMC1551946.

18. Forno, E., & Celedon, J. C. *Curr Opin Allergy Clin Immunol.* 2009. PMID: 19326508

19. Barnett ML, Sommers BD. A National Survey of Medicaid Beneficiaries' Experiences and Satisfaction With Health Care. JAMA Intern Med. 2017 Sep 1;177(9):1378-1381. doi: 10.1001/jamainternmed.2017.3174. Erratum in: JAMA Intern Med. 2017 Sep 1;177(9):1399. doi: 10.1001/jamainternmed.2017.4439. Erratum in: JAMA Intern Med. 2017 Sep 1;177(9):1399. doi: 10.1001/jamainternmed.2017.5056. PMID: 28692734; PMCID: PMC5818833.

20. Roosa Tikkanen and Melinda K. Abrams, U.S. Health Care from a Global Perspective, 2019: Higher Spending, Worse Outcomes? (Commonwealth Fund, Jan. 2020).

21. Aboulenein, Ahmed. U.S. Healthcare Spending Rises to $4.8 trillion in 2023, Outpacing GDP. Accessed at https://www.reuters.com/business/healthcare-pharmaceuticals/us-healthcare-spending-rises-48-trillion-2023-outpacing-gdp-2024-06-12/#:~:text=Medicare%20spending%20is%20project-ed%20to,2023%20and%20%2415%2C074%20in%202024

22. Deutsch, A.L. and Boyle, M.J. The 5 Industries Driving the U.S. Economy. https://www.investopedia.com/articles/investing/042915/5-industries-driving-us-economy.asp

23. Patel, N. and Singhal, S. What to Expect in US Healthcare in 2024 and Beyond. Accessed at https://www.mckinsey.com/industries/healthcare/our-insights/what-to-expect-in-us-healthcare-in-2024-and-beyond#/

24. Center for Health Workforce Studies. "Health Care Employment Projections, 2016-2026: An Analysis of Bureau of Labor Statistics Projections by Setting and by Occupation," Pages 2-3.

25. U.S. Bureau of Labor Statistics. "Projections overview and highlights, 2016–26."

26. Roosa Tikkanen and Melinda K. Abrams, U.S. Health Care from a Global Perspective, 2019: Higher Spending, Worse Outcomes? (Commonwealth Fund, Jan. 2020).

27. Measuring Overall Health System Performance for 191 Countries. Ajay Tandon et al. GPE Discussion Paper Series: No. 30 EIP/GPE/EQC World Health Organization

28. These Countries Have the Most Well-Developed Public Health Systems – CEO Magazine. Available at https://www.usnews.com/news/best-countries/rankings/well-developed-public-health-system

29. Revealed: Countries with the Best Health Care Systems – CEOWORLD Magazine. Available at https://ceoworld.biz/2024/04/02/countries-with-the-best-health-care-systems-2024/

30. The Legatum Prosperity Index 2023. Available at https://www.prosperity.com/rankings

31. Mokdad AH, Marks JS, Stroup DF, Gerberding JL. Actual causes of death in the United States, 2000. Journal of the American Medical Association. 2004;291(10):1238–1245. [PubMed]

32. The Impact of Chronic Underfunding on America's Public Health System: Trends, Risk, and Recommendations, 2020. Trust for America's Health, April 2020.

33. 2024 Edelman Trust Barometer. Accessed at https://www.edelman.com/trust/2024/trust-barometer/special-report-health?utm_campaign=2024%20Trust%20and%20Health&utm_source=media&utm_content=hub#download

34. The Impact of Chronic Underfunding on America's Public Health System: Trends, Risk, and Recommendations, 2020. Trust for America's Health, April 2020.

35. Brousselle A, Benmarhnia T, Benhadj L. What are the benefits and risks of using return on investment to defend public health programs? Prev Med Rep. 2016 Jan 19;3:135-8. doi: 10.1016/j.pmedr.2015.11.015. PMID: 27419005; PMCID: PMC4929139.

36. Dement, John M., Carol Epling, Julie Joyner, and Kyle Cavanaugh. "Impacts of workplace health promotion

and wellness programs on health care utilization and costs: results from an academic workplace." *Journal of Occupational and Environmental Medicine* 57, no. 11 (2015): 1159-1169.

37. Berry, Leonard L. et al. What's the Hard Return on Employee Wellness Programs? Harvard Business Review, Dec. 2010

38. New Mental Health Cost Calculator Shows Why Investing in Mental Health is Good for Business, May 2021. Accessed at https://www.nsc.org/newsroom/new-mental-health-cost-calculator-demonstrates-why

39. Levi, J. et al. Prevention for a Healthier America: Investments in Disease Prevention Yield Significant Savings, Stronger Communities. Trust for America's Health, Feb. 2009. Accessed at https://www.tfah.org

40. Institute of Medicine (US) Roundtable on Evidence-Based Medicine; Yong PL, Saunders RS, Olsen LA, editors. The Healthcare Imperative: Lowering Costs and Improving Outcomes: Workshop Series Summary. Washington (DC): National Academies Press (US); 2010. 6, Missed Prevention Opportunities. Available from: https://www.ncbi.nlm.nih.gov/sites/books/NBK53914/

41. Maciosek MV, Edwards NM, Coffield AB, Flottemesch TJ, Nelson WW, Goodman MJ, Solberg LI. Priorities among effective clinical preventive services: Methods. American Journal of Preventive Medicine. 2006;31(1):90–96.

42. PriceWaterhouseCoopers. The Price of Excess: Identifying Waste in Healthcare Spending. 2008. [accessed July 10, 2024]. http://www.pwc.com/us/en/healthcare/publications/the-price-of-excess.html

43. Cairns C, Kang K. National Hospital Ambulatory Medical Care Survey: 2021 emergency department summary tables. Available from: https://ftp.cdc.gov/pub/Health_Statistics/NCHS/ Dataset_Documentation/NHAMCS/doc21-ed-508.pdf.

44. U.S. Department of Health and Human Services Guidance Portal. Accessed at https://www.hhs.gov/guidance/document/reducing-nonurgent-use-emergency-departments-and-improving-appropriate-care-appropriate

45. GlobalData Plc. *The Complexities of Physician Supply and Demand: Projections from 2021 to 2036.* Washington, DC: AAMC; 2024.

46. Garcia et al. 2010. Emergency Department Visitors and Visits: Who Used the Emergency Room in 2007? CDC, NCHS Data Brief No 38.

47. Gelles-Watnick, R. Americans' Use of Mobile Technology and Home Broadband. January 31, 2024. Accessed at https://pewrsr.ch/49i9IFc

48. Illinois Department of Healthcare and Family Services. *Detailed Managed Care Enrollment, 2024.* Accessed at: https://hfs.illinois.gov/info/factsfigures/detailedmanagedcareenrollment.html

49. Gov. J.B. Pritzker, *Illinois State Budget, Fiscal Year 2025.* Accessed at https://www2.illinois.gov/sites/budget/Pages/default.aspx

50. Vivian Ho, Leanne Metcalfe, Cedric Dark, Lan Vu, Ellerle Weber, George Shelton, and Howard Underwood, "Comparing Utilization and Costs of Care in Freestanding Emergency Departments, Hospital Emergency Departments, and Urgent Care Centers," Annals of Emergency Medicine, February 2017. http://www.annemergmed.com/article/S0196-0644(16)31522-0/pdf

51. Durand AC, Gentile S, Devictor B, et al. ED patients: how nonurgent are they? Systematic review of the emergency medicine literature. Am J Emerg Med. 2011;29:333–345.

52. Premier, Ready, Risk, Reward: Improving Care for Patients with Chronic Conditions (2019).

53. Chou, S-C. et al. Insurance Status and Access to Urgent Primary Care Follow-Up After an Emergency Department Visit in 2016. Ann Emerg Med. 2018;74:487-496.

JEFFREY EMERY STERLING, MD, MPH
SIMPCO PRESIDENT AND CEO

Dr. Jeffrey Sterling is a global leader and in community healthcare, organizational operations, and efficiency. His businesses have created solutions in over three dozen states and countries on five continents. **Sterling Initiatives** is an international healthcare consulting and implementation firm that provides entities with clinical, operational, and financial best practices. **SIMPCO** is America's first managed preventive health organization that, in 2022, successfully steered passage of a $300 million budget item by the State of Illinois to implement health prevention and promotional efforts. **SI Medical Supply** is an international medical, surgical and PPE equipment company. **72 Hours Life** is a personal and professional lifestyle management initiative that teaches efficiency as a means of improving quality of life and business productivity. **SI-STEMS** is a hospitalist and emergency physician staffing company. **www.AskSterlingMD.com** is an online preventive care and urgent care medical service. Dr. Sterling is the author of the popular healthcare blog, 'Straight, No Chaser' and the books *Behind the Curtain: A Peek at Life from within the ER*; *There Are 72 Hours in a Day: Using Efficiency to Better Enjoy Every Part of Your Life*; *The 72 Hours in a Day Workbook*; *Voices and Visions: The Evolution of the Black Experience at Northwestern University*; *Straight, No Chaser Health: Empowering You for Better Health and a Longer Life*; *Learning to Care, Learning to Lead – The History of the Student National Medical Association*; and *Modern Healthcare Heroes – The Legacy of the Student National Medical Association*. Dr.

Sterling currently serves as the first Surgeon General of Alpha Phi Alpha Fraternity, Inc. and as Chairman of both the National Black Chamber of Commerce and the Illinois State Black Chamber of Commerce's Healthcare Committees. Additionally,

- Dr. Sterling has served as CEO, Senior VP, Corporate Medical Officer, National Physician Practice Director, and Regional Medical Director for various health care contract management groups, Medical Director for 17 Emergency Medical System units and Home Health Companies.
- Dr. Sterling has served as Chairman and/or Medical Director of the Departments of Emergency Medicine for over 30 hospitals, including the following Level I Trauma Emergency Departments:
- John Peter Smith Health Network (JPS) in Fort Worth, TX
- Prince George's Hospital Center, Cheverly, Maryland (Metro Washington, D.C.)
- St. Joseph Regional Medical Center, Milwaukee, WI
- Dr. Sterling founded DFW Urgent Care, a series of award-winning urgent care centers in Texas, New York, and California that provide quality, equivalent, cost-effective care alternatives to hospital emergency rooms.
- Dr. Sterling founded the Minority Association of Pre-health Students, a national organization of premedical and other health career aspirants with chapters in over 300 colleges nationally.
- Dr. Sterling was the founding Medical Director for the JPS Health Network Sexual Assault Nurse Examiner (SANE) program and created the first

SANE program in the state of Connecticut at Connecticut Children's Medical Center.

- Dr. Sterling served as President of the Northwestern University Black Alumni Association, representing over 4500 national alumni. He founded Northwestern's Archive of the Black Experience and authored *Voices and Visions: The Evolution of the Black Experience* at *Northwestern University*, which is the only telling of the 145-year history of Blacks at NU. He steered and served as Executive Director of the documentary *The Takeover: The Revolution of the Black Experience at Northwestern University*.

Dr. Sterling has degrees from Northwestern, The Harvard School of Public Health (Health Policy & Management), and the University of Illinois College of Medicine. He completed his Emergency Medicine Residency at Chicago's Stroger (Cook County) Hospital. He received executive education from Dartmouth College's Tuck School of Business.

Dr. Sterling is a speaker in high demand on topics of Medicine, Health Care and Public Health, having delivered over one thousand lectures nationally. He is a regular on various television and radio shows nationally, including Chicago's WGN-TV.

CAROL L. ADAMS, PH.D
SIMPCO CHIEF COMMUNITY
ENGAGEMENT OFFICER

Carol L. Adams, Ph.D., is an applied sociologist, educator, and human services administrator with a distinguished career in public service and a reputation as a change agent. Known for the creation of successful social and community economic development models, her work has taken her from theory to practice and, literally, from the academy to the streets. Having served as the Director of African American Studies at one University and a tenured professor in the School of Education at another, Adams is known for transformational work in challenging environments.

Adams was the first social scientist to serve as Director of the Chicago Housing Authority's Department of Resident Services and Programs. At that time, the CHA was one of the nation's largest public housing developments and ranked among the lowest by the US Department of Housing and Urban Development. During her tenure, Adams' Department was rated 10 (the highest possible rank), and her programs won countless awards in critical areas such as violence reduction, substance abuse treatment and prevention, teen pregnancy, and youth services.

As Secretary of Human Services for the state of Illinois, Adams managed a staff of 15,000 and a budget of over $6 Billion. This mega-agency resulted from the merger of six previously separate departments – Mental Health, Substance Abuse, Community Health and Prevention, Rehabilitation Services, Developmental Disabilities, and Clinical Administration and Program Support. Child Care, Welfare to Work, Prisoner Re-entry, the Food Stamp program and Immigrant and Refugee Services were also a part of the scope of services. Dr. Adams propelled the integration of these once disparate entities into a unified whole and introduced the use of technology to improve service delivery through an innovative initiative called "Online Not In Line." This revolutionary shift made it possible for citizens to access needed services without having to come into offices physically and spend hours waiting in line for assistance. The agency also provided support to the African Association of Chicago, the Continental African Chamber of Commerce, and the Africa International House.

A common thread throughout her remarkable career has been her dedication to Africa and the African Diaspora. As President of the DuSable Museum of African American History, Adams hosted heads of State, provided a venue for conferences and business delegations and mounted exhibitions celebrating the heritage and legacy of Africans throughout the world. A listing of her international engagements includes the following:

<u>Consulting:</u>

- JAMAICA: Evaluation of the Voluntary Organization for the Upliftment of Children (VOUCH) for the US Agency for International Development
- KENYA: Travel and Tourism Marketing campaign for a Kenyan travel agency
- USA: Developed "Teaching About Africa" curriculum for the Chicago Public Schools with Dr. Chernoh Sesay of Chicago State University
- ABIJAN: Fundraising consultant for Presidential candidate
- GHANA: Consultant on Maternal and Child Health
- SOUTH AFRICA: Fundraiser for Shared Interest
- BENIN: Developed and implemented itinerary for delegation of President Boni Yayi
- USA: Resource development for Africa International House

<u>Delegations</u>

- UNITED NATIONS: Member of delegation invited by Kofi Annan to discuss fostering relationships between African Americans and the United Nations
- UGANDA: Member of a trade mission organized by the Africa-USA Chamber of Commerce and the Global Integrated Development Group

- BRAZIL: International cultural exchange sponsored by the National Conference of Artists
- SENEGAL: Hosted President and delegation at the DuSable Museum of African American History
- GHANA: West African connections tour and conference, University of Ghana at Legon, organized by the Congress on Racial Equality
- SOUTH AFRICA: Represented the state of Illinois in a humanitarian mission on HIV/AIDS
- BRAZIL: Organizer of Brazil Cultural Tour for Kennedy-King College
- ZIMBABWE: Delegate on International Business trade mission
- MEXICO: Organizer of the tour to African villages in Mexico
- CUBA: Organizer of cross-cultural, museum exchange tour by DuSable Museum of African American History

NIVA LUBIN-JOHNSON, M.D., FACP
SIMPCO CHIEF HEALTH AND MEDICAL OFFICER

A dedicated physician, Dr. Niva Lubin-Johnson, has been an advocate of quality health care for all, especially the underserved and underrepresented. She was installed as President of the National Medical Association (NMA) on August 14, 2018, and has been an active member of the NMA for over thirty (30) years. In its' 125-year history, Dr. Lubin-Johnson was only the third person and the first female to serve as President, Speaker, and Chair of the Board of Trustees.

Dr. Lubin-Johnson received her B.S. Degree in Pharmacy from Creighton University and her medical degree from Southern Illinois University School of Medicine, where she was distinguished as a member of the last class to finish within a three-year time frame. Dr. Lubin-Johnson completed her Internal Medicine residency at St. Joseph's Hospital, Chicago, and was in private practice for 29 years (in the neighborhood where she grew up and currently resides). She was a senior attending physician at Mercy Hospital and Medical Center; after 25 years as an Associate Attending, she is now an Honorary medical staff member at Advocate Trinity Hospital and a clinical instructor at the University of Illinois. Dr. Lubin-Johnson has participated on several boards and committees at both hospitals, including the Mercy Hospital Executive Medical Board, Advocate-Trinity Physician Hospital Organization Board and the Trinity Medical Staff Medical Executive Committee, currently as Treasurer. She has served for 14 years on the Board of the Independent Physicians at Mercy, an IPA, and currently as Vice-Chair.

She is the Medical Director at Oak Brook Treatment Center, a Methadone Treatment Clinic; Medical Officer of the Day at McFarland Mental Health Residential Center, Springfield, Illinois; and Chief Health Officer of SIMPCO Solutions.

Dr. Lubin-Johnson is a member of the American Medical Association (AMA) and a fellow of the American College of Physicians. She served on the AMA Minority Affairs Section Governing Council from 2010-2017, including 2 as Chair. As Governing Council Chair, she was an Alternate Delegate to the AMA House of Delegates and a member of the AMA/NMA Commission to End Health Care Disparities and its' Diabetes/Hypertension Committee. Now serving on the AMA Women's Physician Governing Council until 2021 and Chair 2019-2021. Other professional memberships and responsibilities include Life Member Student National Medical Association, Trustee, Chicago Medical Society and Delegate to the House of Delegates, member of the Council of Government Affairs, Illinois State Medical Society and Alternate Delegate to the AMA House of Delegates for the Illinois Medical Society. She has served on the Nominating Committee for the Cook County Health System Board for 10 years and is now Chair. In 2017, Dr. Lubin-Johnson was selected to be one of the founding advisory members of TimesUp Healthcare, an organization committed to gender equity for all who have careers in the healthcare industry.

Her service has extended beyond the medical community to higher education as a former Trustee and Chair of the Board of Trustees of Chicago State University, a Traditionally Black University that graduates the most African Americans entering medical school in the state of Illinois. Her mother was a triple alum of CSU. As both her parents succumbed to cancer and her brother to complications of diabetes, she believes in the need for self-care, wellness and preventive care to prevent burnout of physicians, and is also laser-focused on doing all she can to increase the numbers of African Americans entering and completing medical school, especially Black men and serves on the National Medical Association Action/Association of American Medical Colleges Action Collaborative to Increase Black Men in Medical School.

She has lectured extensively in many health forums and is the recipient of numerous awards, including the Illinois Committee of Concerned Blacks in Higher Education Trustee Award; Midwest Community Council—Nancy B. Jefferson Community Service Award; Dollars and Sense Magazine Best and Brightest Women in Medicine; the Kizzy Award—Black Women's Hall of Fame Foundation, the Student National Medical Association Award for Leadership and Service, and the Top Ladies of Distinction Orchid Award for Outstanding Women in Medicine. While Chair of the Board of Trustees for NMA, Dr. Lubin-Johnson attended the annual NGO meeting of the United Nations in Paris and traveled to Accra and Kumasi, Ghana, to begin a program providing specialty care to the Ghanaian population.

Dr. Lubin-Johnson is a proud member of Trinity United Church of Christ and a life member of Alpha Kappa Alpha Sorority, Inc.